Crisliane Gomes de Amorim Lima
Denilson Gomes Silva

The drug clonazepam in the context of the Family Health Strategy

Crisliane Gomes de Amorim Lima
Denilson Gomes Silva

The drug clonazepam in the context of the Family Health Strategy

Care in the rational use of medicines and the search for balance in patients treated in primary health care

Imprint

Any brand names and product names mentioned in this book are subject to trademark, brand or patent protection and are trademarks or registered trademarks of their respective holders. The use of brand names, product names, common names, trade names, product descriptions etc. even without a particular marking in this work is in no way to be construed to mean that such names may be regarded as unrestricted in respect of trademark and brand protection legislation and could thus be used by anyone.

Cover image: www.ingimage.com

This book is a translation from the original published under ISBN 978-613-9-70250-3.

Publisher:
Sciencia Scripts
is a trademark of
Dodo Books Indian Ocean Ltd. and OmniScriptum S.R.L publishing group

120 High Road, East Finchley, London, N2 9ED, United Kingdom
Str. Armeneasca 28/1, office 1, Chisinau MD-2012, Republic of Moldova, Europe
Printed at: see last page
ISBN: 978-620-8-18261-8

I dedicate this work to my brother Paulo Sérgio Gomes de Amorim (in memoriam), who taught me to fight for my dreams and to believe in them without ever doubting that they would work out. Who, with his faith, showed me that life is worth living, always encouraging me to fight for my ideals and giving me strength in the most difficult times. And who always remains with me, no longer physically, but in my thoughts and feelings, part of me forever because every dream realised is alive and never dies.

ACKNOWLEDGEMENTS

To God, for the gift of life and for giving me every opportunity to become patient, wise and humble in the face of obstacles.

To my parents Francisco Ferreira de Amorim and Salete Gomes de Amorim, for their unconditional love and for being the true leaders in my life, always present.

To my husband Estevão da Silva Lima, for his constant encouragement, unconditional support and companionship on this journey.

To my siblings, Eliane Maria Amorim da Silva and Paulo Sérgio Gomes de Amorim (in memoriam), for always supporting me in all my choices, for their companionship and friendship.

To my grandmother Rosa Gomes Ferreira (in memoriam), for always giving me strength in difficult times and for her wisdom in the most complicated situations.

To my mother-in-law Geni Brito da Silva, my father-in-law José Osmar Campos Lima and my sister-in-law Raimunda Márcia da Silva Lima, for their constant support and help in the face of so many difficulties that have arisen along the way.

To my dear nephews Milena Amorim da Silva, Maria Irys Amorim da Silva and Antônio Arthur Amorim da Silva, for their pure and true love and the joy they transmit.

To Professor Denilson Gomes, for his understanding, guidance, encouragement, strength, patience and, above all, respect, companionship and friendship, which made it possible to complete this work and build a better pharmaceutical professional.

To the other professors on the Pharmacy course, for the knowledge they imparted on professional aspects and life lessons.

To true friends and close relatives, for their encouragement, constant support, contribution to learning and lasting bonds of friendship.

To my sister Clívia Brito Oliveira (in memoriam), for her affection, for her support in the face of all decisions, for the honour of having taught me what a true childhood friendship was, with great lessons for a lifetime.

To the great team at the Central Pharmacy of the Santa Casa de Misericórdia de Sobral, for their strength, support, patience, lessons learnt and, above all, for the partnership we have built over time.

To the internship preceptors, for the knowledge they passed on and the patience they showed during the internships.

"Dreams are like gods. If you don't believe in them, they cease to exist. "

CICERO

SUMMARY

Mental health proposes a search for an organised form between emotional and rational internal questions. When individuals experience problems with anxiety and insomnia, they may need psychosocial interventions and drugs, especially the clonazepam dispensed by the Family Health Strategy pharmacy. The aim of this study was to describe the profile of clonazepam users in a basic pharmacy of the Family Health Strategy in Sobral-CE. This is a descriptive, documentary, exploratory, cross-sectional field study with a quantitative approach. The research was carried out at the Maria Eglantine Ponte Guimarães Family Health Centre and the sample consisted of 50 users and their respective prescriptions containing the drug clonazepam from June to September 2016. The data was collected using a questionnaire and prescriptions, and the results were organised considering the information and its specificities using tables and graphs, since the consolidated data was entered into the Microsoft Office Excel® 2007 programme. The results show a prevalence of clonazepam users in terms of gender of around 64 per cent female and 36 per cent male. In terms of age, the majority of users were aged between 40 and 69. As for the length of time they had been using the drug, between 1 and 5 years stood out, which accounted for 74 per cent, and was the most frequent. Prolonged treatment with psychotropic drugs can expose patients to greater susceptibility to the development of possible pharmacological interactions of clinical importance. We identified 31 prescriptions for drugs in association with clonazepam, which accounted for 62 per cent, and 19 prescriptions without an association, which accounted for 38 per cent. As for the medical speciality that prescribed the drug clonazepam, 99% of the prescriptions were written by general practitioners and 1% by psychiatrists. As such, the role of pharmacists in primary health care is necessary to reduce the inappropriate use of this drug, seeking to optimise drug therapy and thus promote quality of life for users.

Keywords: Primary Health Care. Anxiolytics. Pharmaceutical care. Mental Health.

CHAPTER 1

INTRODUCTION

Health is an aggregation of the individual's physical, psychological and social well-being, which seeks not only to resolve the problems of illness that affect the individual, but also to balance the individual's body, mind and spirit (ANDRADE; ANDRADE, 2010).

The patient's healthy state is important because it enables them to relate in a collective and structured way to society as a whole, so that in addition to improving their own performance, they can indirectly influence the actions of others (HELOANI; CAPITÂO, 2003; APOSTOLICO et al., 2007).

Public health, and mental health in particular, proposes a search for an organised form between emotional and rational internal questions, in which if there is a balanced association between these two points, the individual will be developing a broader and more complex well-being (SOUZA, 2014).

When individuals experience problems with anxiety and insomnia, their health is affected as a whole, and they may need psychosocial interventions and the use of drugs. Disorders related to anxiety, depression and insomnia are among the most common and most frequent psychiatric disorders in the population, with a lifetime prevalence of 12.5 per cent (GAVIN, 2013).

When analysing these drugs, benzodiazepines (BZDs) are the class of drugs most commonly used to treat anxiety and insomnia. They have a highly selective mechanism of action for gamma aminobutyric acid (GABAa) receptors, which act on inhibitory synaptic transmission throughout the central nervous system, intensifying the stimulation of GABA, thus facilitating the opening of chloride channels activated by GABA (RANG et al., 2011).

The BZD group is made up of a series of drugs, including clonazepam, in which there are variations in terms of half-life, duration of action and therapeutic indications (FORMAN et al., 2014).

According to Nomura et al. (2006), around 2% of adult patients in the United States used prescription BZDs for at least 12 months and around 50% used these drugs for five years or more.

One of the first household surveys carried out in Brazil found that the use of BZDs without a prescription was around 3.3 per cent of those interviewed (ORLANDI; NOTO, 2005).

States such as Ceará, Pará and Roraima have seen an increase in the consumption of clonazepam, but this drug does not appear in the top position on the list of the National System for the Management of Controlled Products - SNGPC (MANGINI, 2013).

Clonazepam is an anxiolytic drug belonging to the BZD class and aims to improve the lives of patients who develop some kind of disorder, such as panic disorder, and is also used in cases of seizures, i.e. for anticonvulsant purposes (TREVOR; WAY, 2010).

The drug clonazepam is widely used by users of the basic pharmacy in the Family Health Strategy, as it is part of the National List of Essential Medicines (RENAME) and the Municipal List of Essential Medicines (REMUME) - Sobral, as it is part of the clinical protocol of the municipality's monthly demand (ARAÚJO et al., 2012).

In the municipality of Sobral, the Central de Abastecimento Farmacêutico (CAF) provides this drug to the Family Health Centres (CSF) and a high level of distribution is suggested (ARAÚJO et al., 2012). It is worth mentioning that the researcher in charge took part in an extension project on mental health in primary health care with the multi-professional team of a CSF and had access to prescriptions for the drug clonazepam.

The continuous frequency of these prescriptions suggests that the drug is being used indiscriminately, which may imply a view of abuse, and so this study is important to verify the profile of users of this drug. It is also interesting to note that the aim of this study is to provide information on the rational use of medication, providing meaningful pharmaceutical care and interdisciplinary interaction with health professionals.

CHAPTER 2

OBJECTIVES

2.1   General Objective

To describe the profile of clonazepam users in a basic pharmacy of the Family Health Strategy in the city of Sobral-CE.

2.2   Specific objectives

- Identify clonazepam users by gender and age;
- To analyse the types of associations with clonazepam in prescriptions;
- Check how long users have been using clonazepam;
- Checking the origin of prescriptions in terms of medical speciality.

CHAPTER 3

THEORETICAL FRAMEWORK

3.1 Conceptions of Anxiety

Anxiety is said to have its origins in the Greek meaning to suffocate, to oppress. Anxiety or even anguish is related to subjective experiences, thus generating a manifestation of symptoms that the body represents (BARROS et al., 2003). Psychosomatic illnesses are characterised by the presence of anxiety as a behavioural factor (SALLES; SILVA, 2012).

As a result, various social situations arise in which people are faced with excessive anxiety, which is defined by a social anxiety disorder (SAD). This means that people are afraid of expressing themselves in an inappropriate way, relating to traits of showing anxiety, anguish and fear caused by the fear of disapproval and criticism that other people may show because of them. Socialising is avoided or maintained with suffering by this type of being, although there is a desire to relate to other people. This leads to fearful behaviour that tends to lead to avoidance of contact, causing damage to the person's life at work, at school and in other usual social relationships (MULULO et al., 2009).

According to Brasil (2008), there are a number of disorders that are related to anxiety, as shown in Table 1 below:

Chart 1: Anxiety-related disorders.

International Classification of Diseases - ICD 10	Disorder	Definition
F40	Phobic-anxiety disorders	These are disorders where anxiety arises essentiallyor exclusively in situationsniti damente deter mined appear to be in no danger at all. They are situations endured with fear.
F40. 0	Now phobia	It's a disorder that indicates a

			fear of leaving home, of meeting many people, of being in public places or even of travelling somewhere by train or plane alone. Panic disorder also appears, which is the presence of anxiety.
F40. 1		Social phobias	Fear of exposing oneself in social situations and fear of what other people will think. Social neurosis.
F40. 2		Specific (isolated) phobias	Fear of certain animals, thunder, the dark, travelling and the sight of blood. It can also trigger a state of social phobia or panic.
F40. 8		Other phobic-anxious disorders	Phobic state and anxiety.
F40. 9		Unspecified phobic-anxiety disorder	SOE phobic state; SOE phobia.
F41		Other anxiety disorders	A type of disorder that occurs due to the presence of anxiety that arises from something non-specific and can be accompanied by obsessive or depressive symptoms.
F41. 0		Panic disorder (paroxysmal episodic anxiety)	This disorder mainly includes severe anxiety attacks and is therefore unpredictable.
F41.1		Generalised anxiety	In this disorder, the episode occurs in a non-exclusive way, it's something that changes. Persistent nervousness.
F41.2		Mixed anxiety and depressive disorder	It is a disorder in which there is a mixture of symptoms of anxiety and depression.

		However diagnosed in isolation.
F 41.3	Other mixed anxiety disorders	These are disorders in which the characteristics are related to other disorders. Not being justified diagnosis in the face of an isolated symptom.
F41.8	Other specified anxiety disorders	Anguish hysteria.
F 41.9	Non-anxiety disorder specified	Anxiety.

Source: BRASIL, 2008.

3.2 Physiopathology of Anxiety

Anxiety as visualised by biology is directed by the performance of the brain, which acts with environmental perceptions, interconnecting with events that reinforce or lead to situations of flight, where these perceptions result in storage memories for an understanding of defence data where fight and flight are part of the context. Different connections occur in this system where gabaergic, serotoninergic, dopaminergic and other pathways are present (BERNIK et al., 1999).

Anxiety is said to be a state in which the hypothalamic-pituitary-adrenal axis is activated, as well as the sympathetic-adrenal axis, and can develop characteristics such as tachycardia, dry mouth, excessive sweating, hypertension, insomnia, anguish and fears (GRAEFF, 2007; COGHI; COGHI, 2013).

It is understood that there has been an evolution in the understanding of the organisation of neural systems in the face of anxiety. Studies have shown that behaviour related to fear and threat stimuli is directly related to defence and is in turn intertwined with states of anxiety, whereby the cerebral defence system and the behavioural inhibition system are involved in anxiety (HETEM; GRAEFF, 2012).

3.3 Treatment with Anxiolytics

According to Carvalho and Dimenstein (2004), the use of anxiolytics is a problem that has taken on great dimensions, thus becoming a concern in the area of public health, due to the relationship of dependence as a result of the indiscriminate administration of these drugs.

These drugs can cause serious social problems and personal problems for individuals who become accustomed to their use and in turn become a common part of everyday life. These drugs, which are known to calm, tranquillise and even sedate, are called anxiolytics, acting through the Central Nervous System (CNS), providing the patient with a selective action on their anxiety.

This situation of dependence is related to issues of escaping from social life and the problems it can bring, family friction or even stressful situations in the workplace. It was because of this that the use of BZDs was shown to be safe and so a culture of lack of responsibility was created through their prescription, dispensation and administration. In the same vein, BZDs should be taken for a certain period of time, which is said to be between two and four months, but it can be seen that treatment varies over a longer period of time, where it is no longer something for specific purposes but is treated as an essential and necessary medication, as in the case of anxiety-related problems (CARVALHO; DIMENSTEIN, 2004).

Rang et al. (2011), can be placed as a classification of drug groups of this function in Table 2 below:

Table 2: Main classes of anxiolytics.

Classification of drugs	
Benzodiazepines	Used as anxiolytic and hypnotic agents.
Buspirone	Used as a serotonin 1A receptor agonist, with an anxiolytic function, but its sedative effect is not noted.
Beta adrenergic receptor antagonists (propranolol)	Used to treat anxiety when symptoms such as sweating, tremor and tachycardia occur. Good results when peripheral sympathetic responses are blocked rather than central effects.
Zolpidem	Used in a similar way to BZDs, it is chemically distinct, has a hypnotic function and is not an important anxiolytic.
Barbiturates	Their uses have become obsolete as they have been replaced by BZDs, which now have greater specificity as anaesthetics and antiepileptics.
Various drugs (meprobamate, chloral hydrate and methaqualone)	They are no longer recommended for use, but they are used on occasion. It's interesting to note that diphenhydramine (a sedative antihistamine) is sometimes used as a hypnotic, especially for children.

Source: RANG et al., 2011.

3. 4Benzodiazepines

Anxiolytic and hypnotic drugs that have a high therapeutic index and great effect properties are known as BZDs, which also have anticonvulsant purposes (MIHIC; HARRIS, 2012). It is possible to report that the use of this class of drugs is widespread, as it ranges from developing countries to the most developed (HUF; LOPES; ROZENFELD, 2000; DIÉYE, 2006).

Since the 1980s, public health problems have been detected in Chile with regard to the inappropriate use of BZDs, as the rate of consumption was not only high, but sometimes occurred without a medical indication to justify it (GALLEGUILLOS et al., 2003).

Brasil (2006), quoted by Filho (2011), says that BZDs act on the central nervous system, which can lead to changes in psychomotor and cognitive expression in the individual's structure. They have therapeutic effects such as muscle relaxation, hypnosis and sedation. They are also indicated in clinical practice for anxiety, sleep disorders, convulsions and involuntary muscle spasms.

It is known that the use of this class of drugs causes high levels of tolerance and dependence, so it is also necessary to increase the dose of the drug so that it can perform the same therapeutic result as before, and it should not be discontinued at random, since it can cause symptoms and signs that are the opposite of what is expected from this type of drug. Studies have shown that the long-term use of BZD's leads to a decrease in the activity of thinking and interpreting in the elderly with greater emphasis, further amplifying the natural absence of function at this stage of life (BICCA; ARGIMON, 2008). Studies also indicate that there is a strong relationship between age and gender with the consumption of BZDs (ALVARENGA et al., 2008; SILVA; BATISTA; ASSIS, 2013).

In Brazil, there are factors that contribute even more to the rampant use of psychotropic medication, as it is clear that free distribution through government programmes is a fact, without there being any measures to actually control access, thus making it easier to obtain medication (CRUZ et al., 2006).

It can be seen that when prescriptions are misused, the flow of BZDs increases even more, and they end up becoming chronic. A large proportion of patients use prescriptions from general practitioners or various specialities, not just psychiatrists, leading to various future problems, including long-term use of these medications and dependence (ORLANDI; NOTO, 2005).

Rang et al. (2011) describes the main BZDs in Table 3 below:

Table 3: Characteristics of benzodiazepines.

Medicines	Duration of Action	Use of the drug
Clonazepam	Long	Anticonvulsants anxiolytic.
Flurazepam	Long	Anxiolytic.
Diazepam Chlordiazepoxide	Long	Anxiolytic, relaxing muscle.
		0 diazepam is used

		intravenously with the function of anticonvulsant.
Nitrazepam	Average	Anxiolytic and hypnotic.
Alprazolam	Average	Antidepressant anxiolytic.
Lormetazepam Temazepam Oxazepam Lorazepam	Short	Hypnotic and anxiolytic.
Zolpidem	Ultracurta	Hypnotic.
Triazolam Midazolam	Ultracurta	Hypnotic. Midazolam is used as an anaesthetic intravenously.

Source: RANG et al., 2011.

3.5 Pharmacotherapy of Clonazepam

The drug clonazepam, which belongs to the BZD class, has a number of properties including anticonvulsant action, sedation, tranquillisation and muscle relaxation (MIHIC; HARRIS, 2012). It is used alone or as an aid in epileptic seizures, absence, partial, generalised and infantile spasms. It is also used for anxiety disorders, panic disorder, mood disorders, social phobia, some psychotic syndromes, vertigo, balance disorders, nausea followed by vomiting with pre-syncope or syncope, falls, tinnitus and hearing disorders (GREENBLATT et al., 2005; BRASIL, 2013a).

Clonazepam is derived from 7-nitrobenzodiazepine (KOROLKOVAS; BURCKHALTER, 2013). One of its functions is mild inhibition of the central nervous system (CHAUHAN et al., 2000). Its chemical formula is 5-(o-chlorophenyl)-1,3-dihydro-7-nitro-2H-1,4-benzodiazepine-2-one, with the molecular formula $C_{15}H_{10}ClN_3O_3$, molecular weight 315.72 g/mol, it is a crystalline powder with a light yellow colour, has a fast smell, is poorly soluble in alcohol, ether and soluble in acetone and chloroform (SONG; ZHANG; KOHLHOF, 1996; CAVEDAL, 2014). It is active as a CNS depressant, and can act with something as simple as sedation or hypnosis, thus varying the dosage. It is a stimulator of GABA receptors, has rapid absorption if administered orally, where oral bioavailability is around ninety per cent and maximum concentration occurs in 1 to 4 hours (RANG et al., 2011). Its main metabolite is 7- aminoclonazepam - 7 aclo (CHÈZE; VILLAIN; PÉPIN, 2004).

Absorption takes place in the gastrointestinal tract, then it is rapidly distributed to various organs and tissues in the body, brain structures and has a binding to plasma proteins of 85%, it also has a high rate of metabolisation, with less than 2% being eliminated in the urine in an unchanged way, elimination is around 30 to 40 hours (FORMAN et al., 2014).

According to Cavedal (2014), there are several adverse reactions to the use of clonazepam, such as disorders of the immune system that include some cases of anaphylaxis and allergic reactions, psychiatric disorders with the presence of a state of confusion, restlessness and even loss of libido, disorders of the nervous system that can lead to dizziness, headaches, eye disorders such as diplopia, respiratory system disorders such as respiratory depression, skin and subcutaneous tissue disorders such as pruritus, pigmentation changes, skeletal muscle disorders such as muscle weakness, urinary and kidney disorders such as urinary incontinence, reproductive system disorders such as erectile dysfunction.

It is included in the list of the National List of Essential Medicines (RENAME), where it is formulated as a 2.5 mg/ml oral solution, thus forming part of pharmaceutical assistance (BRASIL, 2013b).

According to Ordinance no. 344/98 - SVS/MS, of 12 May 1998, the substance clonazepam is subject to special control, as it is part of the definition of psychotropic substances, which appears on list B1, requiring the notification of a B prescription (BRASIL, 1998). ANVISA states that clonazepam should be used while fasting and with care and attention to the dose (BRASIL, 2013c; BRASIL, 2015).

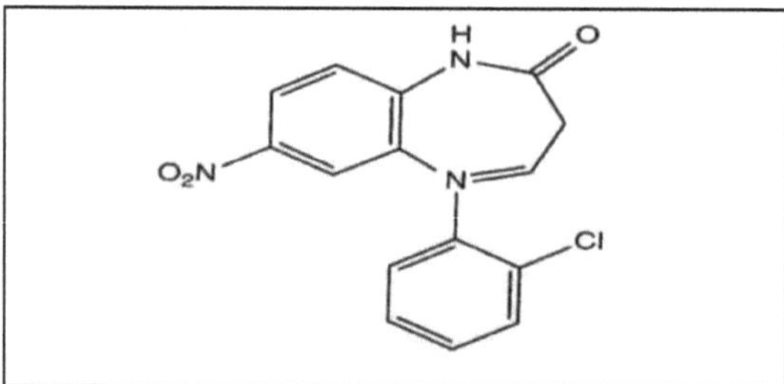

Figure 1: Chemical structure of clonazepam.
Source: KOROLKOVAS; BURCKHALTER, 2013.

3.   6Pharmaceutical Care   in Primary Care and Mental Health

When the Unified Health System (Sistema Único de Saúde - SUS) came into being, there were also adequate subsidies for health in an expanded form. Within this context, pharmaceutical services are responsible for promoting health and avoiding problems with the possible inappropriate use of drugs. This concern could be resolved with the active participation of a professional pharmacist, who becomes fundamental within this policy, given that there are studies that show that there is little recruitment of pharmacists for the SUS, and that they can also work in service management, clinical analyses and health surveillance (BANHOS, 2006; LENZI; GARCIA; PONTAROLO, 2011).

The search for quality in healthcare focuses on the degree of professional merit, efficiency and effectiveness in relation to the resources made available, concern for the patient's condition, satisfaction and positive effects for organised and balanced health (ARAÚJO et al., 2008).

This is the context of Primary Health Care (PHC), which is a form of strategy and organisation for something more elaborate in terms of health care, focusing on a continuous and systematised way of meeting the needs of the population, linking promotion, protection and prevention actions, making it possible for pharmacists to be part of this process, since pharmaceutical care is also part of the SUS. The National Medicines Policy (Política Nacional de Medicamentos - PNM) defined pharmaceutical care activities as a group of activities related to medicines, aimed at supporting a community's health actions (MARGONATO, 2006). The term Pharmaceutical Services involves comprehensive, multi-professional and intersectoral activities, the object of which is the organisation of actions and services focused on medicines in their various dimensions, with an emphasis on the relationship with the patient and a vision of health promotion (REIS, et al., 2003). It was in 2004 that the National Health Council published the National Pharmaceutical Care Policy (PNAF), which reinforces the idea that pharmaceutical care should be characterised as part of individual or collective health care, with medicines as essential, as access must be guaranteed with rational use (VIEIRA, 2010).

The same concept is also applied to Mental Health, which focuses on the balance between mind and body, uniting to create a good harmony in order to intervene in a healthy way when living in contact with the world. Thus, the Brazilian psychiatric reform also required changes in pharmaceutical care, conceived as a set of actions and services aimed at ensuring comprehensive therapeutic care, health promotion and recovery, including research activities and the pharmaceutical care cycle. They are understood as essential health supplies that must be able to be used rationally. CAPS should therefore be a reference point for dispensing mental health medicines. However, the Family Health Strategy takes on responsibility in this process, providing adequate staff to assist these users, in order to meet the different needs and objectives of the mental health and pharmaceutical assistance policy, especially with regard to the availability, dispensation and promotion of the rational use of medicines (BRASIL, 2004).

In this way, there are still spaces in the process of reorienting pharmaceutical care that problematise the logic of the activities, which in turn affect the health of users with mental illnesses. And it is in this reality that it is necessary to take a new look at the services that have been developed in order to guarantee better structured pharmaceutical care for these users, since the rational use of medicines is fundamental in the treatment of mental disorders (ALENCAR; CAVALCANTE;

ALENCAR, 2012).

The pharmacist's role in pharmaceutical care must be in harmony with what users need in order to be able to obtain the drugs necessary for the individual's therapy. Standardising, acquiring and distributing these drugs allows for administrative rationality and patient health safety (REIS et al., 2003; MESTRINER, 2003).

Dispensing is a function in which there must be a search for continuous knowledge, because the rational use of medicines becomes better founded when the professional has extensive knowledge and can pass this on to the client when dispensing the medicines, at which point all doubts are removed and successful pharmacotherapy is expected (LENZI; GARCIA; PONTAROLO, 2011).

Pharmaceutical care is the key point in the relationship between professional and patient, with respect and quality in what is offered (OLIVEIRA; ASSIS; BARBONI, 2010). The rational use of medicines is also emphasised as one of the concerns where the pharmacist must be able to solve the client's needs (FIRMINO et al., 2012).

CHAPTER 4

METHODOLOGY

4.1 Type of Study

This is a descriptive field study, as well as a documentary, exploratory, cross-sectional study with a predominantly quantitative approach.

According to Marconi and Lakatos (2010), in descriptive research, the facts are observed, recorded, analysed, classified and interpreted, without the researcher interfering in them.

Documentary research is a source of data collection that is restricted to documents, whether written or not, and is characterised as primary sources. It can be carried out at the time the action or phenomenon takes place or afterwards (MARCONI; LAKATOS, 2010).

Exploratory research is something that has not been extensively investigated. When an exploratory study is finalised, the researcher will be more aware of the subject and able to develop hypotheses based on the results obtained in the study (GIL, 2011).

A cross-sectional study makes use of exposing something relatively constant over time and the effect of this information on the research (HOCHMAN et al., 2005).

In the quantitative approach, it is necessary to organise the preparation of documents, interviews, questionnaires, statistical values, observation and conclusions in order to carry out the research properly (SEVERINO, 2007).

4.2 Place of Study and Period

The research took place between June and September 2016 at the Maria Eglantine Ponte Guimarães Family Health Centre (FHC), which is located on Travessa Dom Expedito and was given this name on 20 June 2001. It is better known as the Dom Expedito CSF, which covers the Dom Expedito and Santo Antonio neighbourhoods in the city of Sobral - Ceará.

The Dom Expedito CSF is made up of: 05 Nurses; 02 Doctors; 02 Dentists; 10 Community Health Agents; 03 Nursing Technicians; 02 Oral Health Technicians; 06 Administrative Agents; 05 professionals (Psychologist, Nutritionist, Physiotherapist, Social Worker and Physical Educator) who are part of the Family Health Support Centre (NASF); 06 professionals from the Multiprofessional Residency in Family Health (Psychologist, Nutritionist, Physiotherapist, Social Worker, Pharmacist and Physical Educator); 04 General Services Assistants; 05 Watchmen.

Pharmacists work in three different ways within the primary health care service: as participants in multi-professional health residency programmes, NASF and as pharmacists hired by the establishment. In this approach, the resident pharmacist is characterised as being a propagator of the principles and guidelines of the SUS, designed to implant knowledge and be able to have a positive impact on the territory in which they are located, bringing benefits to the population. It is in the NASF that the participation of a team aimed at building a collective intervention and integration is also included, with the aim of acting in an integrated manner and in participation with various health professionals, thus trying to expand user care in the CSF and raise the quality of the pharmacist's performance in patient care. Pharmacists have a very important role to play in a number of situations, in which it is always necessary to take a close look at the situation of individuals who use public health services, and it is in Primary Care that a participatory approach should be developed that links health professionals, users, comprehensive care and the active participation of everyone (MELO et al., 2009; COSTA; RABELO; DE LIMA, 2014).

The services offered at the CSF are: reception and screening; vaccinations; dressings and medication administration; medical and nursing consultations; medication dispensing; mental health care; educational activities; home visits; hypertension and diabetes control; Sexually Transmitted Diseases (STD) treatment; Tuberculosis and Leprosy treatment; monitoring children's development and growth; family planning; prenatal care; breast and gynaecological cancer prevention; registration of families living in the team's area of responsibility; collection for laboratory tests.

The CSF has accessible conditions for carrying out this study, as it is a public body, has a pharmacist (resident) and a flow of around 260 users who are part of Mental Health, which includes the use of the drug clonazepam.

4.3 Population

The population involved in the research is around 4,000 families, with approximately 260 mental health users with some form of mental disorder being monitored, 100 of whom make regular use of clonazepam. The sample was made up of only 50 users who used the drug clonazepam dispensed at the CSF pharmacy in a prospective study.

4.4 Data Collection

The data was collected by means of a questionnaire (APPENDIX B) that was carried out with 50 users and then an assessment of their respective prescriptions available at the study site.

4.5 Inclusion and Exclusion Criteria

The questionnaires and clonazepam prescriptions of users over the age of 18 were entered during the study period. Those who did not meet the above standards were removed.

4.6 Data Analysis and Presentation

The results were organised considering the information and its specificities using tables and graphs, since this is a quantitative survey and the consolidated data was entered into the Microsoft Office Excel® 2007 programme.

4.7 Risks and benefits

The risks of the research were kept to a minimum and, in order to minimise these risks, only information acquired through a questionnaire was used, which the participants felt free to answer, in order to ensure their confidentiality and protection. They were then given access to their prescriptions at the CSF pharmacy. The benefits of the research were to identify the number of users of the drug clonazepam registered at the study site, to monitor the care provided by the pharmacist and the multi-professional team, and to minimise possible difficulties in therapeutic adherence through the integration, collaboration and participation of the multi-professional team.

4.8 Ethical aspects

The research project was appraised by the Scientific Committee of the Health Studies and Research Centre (NEPS) of the Sobral - Ceará Health Department, which issued an authorisation opinion (APPENDIX A) and then the research protocols were completed and submitted to the Brazil Platform, where the project was assessed and approved by the Research Ethics Committee (CEP) of the Vale do Acaraú State University (UVA) in Sobral - Ceará, by means of a substantiated opinion and Certificate of Presentation for Ethical Appraisal - Opinion no.1.579.536 (APPENDIX B).

User data was kept confidential in accordance with Resolution no. 466/12 of the National Health Council (CNS)/Ministry of Health (MS), with its Guidelines and Norms regulating research involving human beings in Brazil (BRASIL, 2013d), which revoked Resolution no. 196/96. Therefore, the participants received adequate information about the research and then signed the Informed Consent Form (ICF) (APPENDIX A).

CHAPTER 5

RESULTS AND DISCUSSION

We identified 50 users who received the drug clonazepam at the pharmacy of the Maria Eglantine Ponte Guimarães CSF in Sobral - CE during the study period, in which various data were analysed, such as: gender, age, length of use of the drug clonazepam, place of consultation, association and origin of the prescription, as shown in the following tables.

Table 1. Representation of males and females in prescriptions filled at the pharmacy of the Maria Eglantine Ponte Guimarães Family Health Centre in Sobral - CE, between June and September 2016.

SEX	NUMBER	PERCENTAGE (%)
FEMALE	32	64
MALE	18	36
TOTAL	50	100

Source: Direct research, 2016.

Table 1 shows the prevalence of female (64%) compared to male (36%) use of the drug clonazepam, which can be explained by the fact that women are more concerned about their health and are more aware of issues related to self-care, as they tend to use health services more often.

Women are more informed about adherence to drug treatments because they are more present in health services and this reflects a natural way for doctors to treat symptoms of depression and anxiety differently between the sexes, detecting these illnesses more easily in women, which results in a greater number of prescriptions for the female sex (LOYOLA; UCHOA; LIMA, 2006).

The possible causes of the higher consumption of psychotropic drugs by women may be related to the following aspects: women's longer life expectancy, the visualisation of more illnesses, the fact that they undergo more tests related to prevention and the greater use, in a way, of health services (MENDONÇA; CARVALHO, 2005).

Table 2. Age range of patients seen and using the drug clonazepam at the pharmacy of the Maria Eglantine Ponte Guimarães Family Health Centre in Sobral - CE, from June to September 2016.

AGE GROUP	NUMBER	PERCENTAGE (%)
18 TO 29 YEARS	8	16
30 TO 39 YEARS	8	16
40 TO 49 YEARS	9	18
50 TO 59 YEARS	10	20
60 TO 69 YEARS	9	18
70 TO 79 YEARS	4	8
80 TO 89 YEARS	2	4
TOTAL	50	100

Source: Direct research, 2016.

Table 2 shows that the majority of patients were aged between 40 and 69. The minimum age observed was 18 and the maximum was 89. This shows that there were variations in the age range, with a prevalence of middle-aged and elderly users.

The profile of users of this type of drug is generally the elderly and other middle-aged individuals, and this is seen as a relevant factor in proving that these patients use this medication not only for the purpose of hypnotic medication and anxiolytic effect respectively, but also to ease situations involving stress, family problems and other health problems (SILVA, 2012).

Other studies have shown that the use of BZDs for long periods of time by the elderly can lead to a greater increase in dependence on substances that affect the CNS, as well as facilitating more exacerbated exposure to falls, respiratory problems and a greater increase in the number of deaths due to sleep apnoea syndrome (DO AMARAL; MACHADO, 2012).

Table 3. Time of use of the drug clonazepam in the pharmacy of the Maria Eglantine Ponte Guimarães CSF Health Centre in Sobral - CE, from June to September 2016.

TIME INTERVAL	NUMBER	PERCENTAGE (%)
LESS THAN 1 YEAR	5	10
BETWEEN 1 AND 5 YEARS	37	74
MORE THAN 5 YEARS	8	16
TOTAL	50	100

Source: Direct research, 2016.

In order to facilitate analysis, the length of use of the medication involved in this study was organised into time intervals, as shown in Table 3. It was observed that the time interval of more than 5 years accounted for 16%, and between 1 and 5 years accounted for 74%, which were the most frequent. There was also a lower frequency of use for less than 1 year, which accounted for 10%.

Prolonged treatment with psychotropic drugs can expose patients to greater susceptibility to the development of possible pharmacological interactions of clinical importance, since during treatment there may be a need to use other drugs (SANTOS et al., 2009).

Prolonged use of high doses of BZDs, especially in primary psychiatric disorders (anxiety, sleep disorders), which require a longer treatment period of 4 to 6 weeks, can lead to tolerance, withdrawal and possibly addiction, as this occurs more easily when high-potency drugs with a short half-life are prescribed.

Thus, it is understood that BZDs should be used for short periods and with greater care from health professionals (CASTRO et al., 2013).

According to Cruz et al. (2006), the use of psychotropic drugs for up to three months presents practically no risk to health; between three and twelve months, the risk increases to 10% to 15% and use for more than twelve months presents a risk of 25% to 40%. It is important to emphasise that users of psychotropic medication should be monitored periodically in order to ensure effective treatment and minimise side effects.

TIPO DE CONSULTA MÉDICA

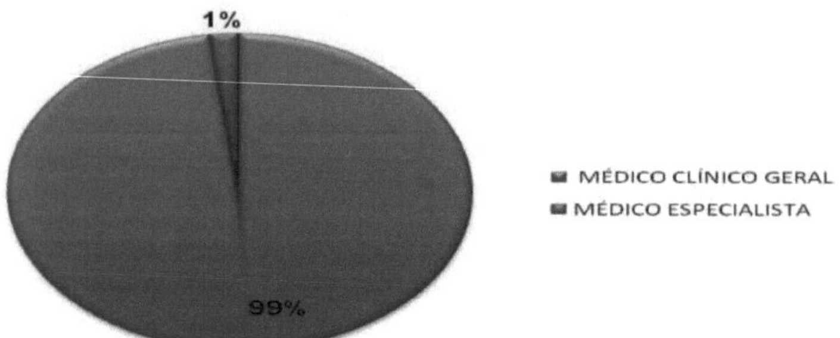

Graph 1. Occurrence of medical prescriptions at the Maria Eglantine Ponte Guimarães Family Health Centre in Sobral - CE, between June and September 2016.
Source: Direct research, 2016.

Graph 1 shows the type of care provided at the CSF, where it can be seen that 49 of the prescriptions were developed by general practitioners, but only 1 was carried out by a specialist (psychiatrist). The general practitioner is usually the first to receive complaints of a psychological or psychosocial nature (NORDON; HUBNER, 2009).

Do Amaral and Machado (2012) report that in this type of situation there are some factors that contribute to a higher prevalence of BZD misuse.

Free distribution through government programmes without actually analysing the patient's real needs, failures that occur when these drugs are dispensed, improper prescriptions in the face of various complaints, and the patient's own lack of knowledge.

With regard to the place of consultation and the medical speciality that prescribes the drug clonazepam, it can be seen that users are not being monitored by specialist doctors. This is justified by the shortage of specialist doctors and the lack of monitoring by the multiprofessional team at the CSF, which could refer these users to the Psychosocial Support Centre (CAPS), so that these users could possibly be more effective in their treatment, improving their quality of life and minimising public health costs.

Table 4 Types of associations with the drug clonazepam found in prescriptions filled at the pharmacy of the Maria Eglantine Ponte Guimarães Family Health Centre in Sobral - CE, between June and September 2016.

TYPE OF ASSOCIATIONS	NUMBER	PERCENTAGE (%)
CLONAZEPAM + HALOPERIDOL	3	6
CLONAZEPAM + CARBAMAZEPINE	5	10

24

CLONAZEPAM + AMITRIPTYLINE	10	20
CLONAZEPAM + FLUOXETINE	10	20
CLONAZEPAM + BIPERIDEN	3	6
NO ASSOCIATION	19	38
TOTAL	50	100

Source: Direct research, 2016.

According to Table 4, 31 prescriptions were identified in association with the drug clonazepam, which represented 62%, further detailed with the respective information below: Clonazepam + Haloperidol drugs, which were found in 6%, Clonazepam + Carbamazepine drugs, which were found in 10%, Clonazepam + Amitriptyline drugs, which were found in 20%, Clonazepam + Fluoxetine drugs, which were found in 20%, Clonazepam + Biperidene drugs, which were found in 6%. Nineteen prescriptions with no association were identified, representing 38 per cent.

Drug interactions are considered to be characteristics of the effects of a drug when administered in association with other drugs, food or other chemical substances, which may or may not interfere with damage to health (ANDRADE; BARRETO, 2014).

Identifying the classes of drugs used is very important, as some drugs have a higher rate of probable drug interactions, especially antidepressants, anticonvulsants and BZDs (SANTOS et al., 2009).

The association between haloperidol and clonazepam was found in three patients, and can result in synergistic effects with neuroleptics, which can increase extrapyramidal reactions, as well as increasing haloperidol levels by 26%; increase the appearance of dizziness and sedation (FONSECA, 2008). Haloperidol can reduce the metabolism and clearance of clonazepam and thus increase serum concentration, resulting in increased effects (TURATTI; MARINI, 2014).

It was noted that BZDs are often combined with antiepileptic drugs, and that the effects of these interactions can lead to respiratory depression and coma. Carbamazepine, observed in association with clonazepam in five prescriptions, reduces the effectiveness of this drug. It acts as an inducer of the CYP3A4 metabolic enzyme and is capable of speeding up the process of biotransformation and elimination of BZDs (FONSECA, 2008; MIHIC; HARRIS, 2012).

Possible drug interactions between BZDs appear in association with antidepressants. Ten associations were found with the tricyclic antidepressant amitriptyline and ten with the selective serotonin reuptake inhibitor fluoxetine. Tricyclics, as well as selective serotonin reuptake inhibitors, inhibit the metabolic enzymes CYP2C19 and CYP3A4, contributing to an increase in plasma levels and the effects of BZDs in the body (MIHIC; HARRIS, 2012). Thus, in relation to the risk exposed to the patient, this association is considered to be of a moderate degree (FONSECA, 2008).

SSRIs are widely prescribed antidepressants because they are less prone to adverse effects than tricyclic antidepressants and monoamine oxidase inhibitors (MAOIs) (REMINGTON, 2012). It is important to emphasise that fluoxetine hydrochloride combined with clonazepam has benefits in terms of its anti-obsessive effect and increased sedation, but can develop memory and psychomotor problems (BARBOZA; SILVA, 2012).

The SSRIs are highlighted in order to find research aimed at finding effective drugs compared to tricyclic antidepressants, but with fewer tolerability and safety problems. There is a high use of fluoxetine hydrochloride, due to the fact that its treatment abandonment rates are lower compared to other antidepressants. When antidepressants are tested by the population, it is only analysed that they have good efficacy, but their side effects change from one drug to another and this is unfortunately not observed as an exclusion criterion at the very first attempt at therapy. Thus, if the least harmful choice is to be made, fluoxetine hydrochloride is the one best suited to the situation (REMINGTON, 2012; CREPALDI, 2013).

Combination therapy of ADT plus BDZ at the start of treatment for anxiety, panic disorder, depression or other co-existing illnesses, increases the potency of the effect of the drugs or even provides control of undesirable pharmacological reactions that only one drug in the therapy would cause. From another angle, drug-drug interactions can be offensive to the patient, causing very serious adverse effects and the cost-benefit ratio is not fundamental in this situation (CAMPIGOTTO et al., 2008; MOJTABAI; OLFSON, 2010).

The association of three prescriptions was found between clonazepam and biperidene, which is characterised as a central anticholinergic, because it is able to block muscarinic receptors at a central and peripheral level and also prevents the reuptake of dopamine by nerve terminals, it is effective in promoting sedation and mental confusion, so it can trigger an increase in the potency of the depressant action of BZDs (SILVA, 2010; MIHIC; HARRIS, 2012).

Prescriptions with combinations need constant attention and care, which includes evaluating the medicines in use and gaining a better knowledge of them, trying to reduce the number of substances used, and controlling and minimising the side effects that may arise during therapy (MIYASAKA; ATALLAH, 2003).

It is in pharmaceutical counselling that we can work on patient adherence to therapy, seeking to inform them of the benefits and risks of the medicines used, avoiding future problems with a correct way of understanding what the therapy of these drugs is and how the patient themselves can help in this training, implying a better quality of care and attention between professional and patient (ALENCAR; NASCIMENTO, 2011).

Pharmacists are trained to attend to patients and assess and guide their pharmacotherapy, which is induced by the doctor, by analysing their need to use medicines and, after finding Drug-Related Problems (DRPs), they must try to work with other health professionals to correct or reduce the possible risks involved in the therapy (OLIVEIRA et al., 2005; NUNES et al., 2008).

CHAPTER 6

FINAL CONSIDERATIONS

More elaborate and time-consuming studies need to be carried out to confirm the various pharmaceutical associations with psychotropic drugs, so that greater care and supervision can be exercised in the dispensing of these drugs, with a view to improving therapy and reducing the costs of public health services.

It's worth pointing out that health professionals need to take a close look at the pharmacist's suggestions for the necessary guidelines that should be passed on to patients when dispensing medicines, especially when it comes to CNS-related substances.

Thus, the role of pharmacists in primary health care is important, whether it's to establish clear procedures for dispensing psychotropic drugs or to introduce continuing education measures for health professionals in order to adequately prepare the multi-professional team. These are fundamental tools in reducing the inappropriate use of these drugs, optimising patients' quality of life and drug therapy.

REFERENCES

ALENCAR, T. O. S.; CAVALCANTE, E. A. B.; ALENCAR, B. R. Assistência farmacêutica e saúde mental no Sistema Único de Saúde. **Revista de Ciências Farmacêuticas Básica e Aplicada**, v. 33, n. 4, p. 489-495, 2012.

ALENCAR, T. O. S.; NASCIMENTO, M. A. Pharmaceutical assistance in the Family Health Programme: encounters and mismatches in the organisational process. **Ciência Saúde coletiva**, v. 16, n. 9, p. 3939-3949, 2011.

ALVARENGA, J. M. et al. Prevalence and sociodemographic characteristics associated with the use of benzodiazepines by community-dwelling elderly: Bambuí project. **Revista Brasileira de Psiquiatria**, v. 30, n. 1, p. 7-11, 2008.

ANDRADE, E. N.; ANDRADE, E. O. OUS and the Brazilian right to health: a reading of its principles, with emphasis on universal coverage. **Revista Bioética**, v. 18, n. 1, p. 61-74, 2010.

ANDRADE, K. V. F.; BARRETO, Z. D. Pharmacoepidemiological profile of potential drug interactions in psychotropic drug prescriptions. **Revista Eletrônica de Farmácia**, v. 11, n. 4, p. 72-85, 2014.

APOSTOLICO, M. R. et al. Contribution of cipesc to the implementation of child health care policies in the municipality of Curitiba, Paraná. **Texto & Contexto - Enfermagem**, v. 16, n. 3, p. 453-462, 2007.

ARAÚJO, A. L. A. et al. Profile of pharmaceutical care in primary care of the Unified Health System. **Ciência & Saúde Coletiva**, v. 13, supl, p. 611-617, 2008.

ARAÚJO, L. L. C. et al. Distribution of antidepressants and benzodiazepines in the family health strategy of Sobral - CE. **Revista de Políticas Públicas - Sobral**, v. 11, n.1, p. 45-54, 2012.

BANHOS, R. M. O. **Implementation of pharmaceutical care in the single health system (SUS) of Alfenas - MG.** 2006. 66f. Course Conclusion Paper (Specialisation in Pharmaceutical Care) - Federal University of Alfenas, Minas Gerais, 2006.

BARBOZA, P. S.; SILVA, D. A. Antidepressant and antipsychotic drugs prescribed at the psychosocial care centre (CAPS) in the municipality of Porciúncula - RJ. **Acta Biomédica Brasiliensia**, v. 3, n. 1, p. 85-97, 2012.

BARROS, A. L. B. L. et al. Anxiety-generating situations and strategies for their control among nurses: a preliminary study. **Revista Latino-Americana de Enfermagem**, v. 11, n. 5, p. 585-592, 2003.

BERNIK, M. A. et al. **Benzodiazepines: four decades of experience.** 4. ed. São Paulo: USP, 1999.

BICCA, M. G.; ARGIMON, I. I. L. Cognitive abilities and use of benzodiazepines in institutionalised elderly women. **Brazilian Journal of Psychiatry**, v. 57, n. 2, p. 133138, 2008.

BRAZIL. Ministry of Health. **Technical Note No. 293/2013**. Brasília, DF, 2013a.

BRAZIL. Ministry of Health. **RENAME: National List of Essential Medicines**. Brasília, DF, 2013b.

BRAZIL. Ministry of Health. Resolution no. 338, of 6th May 2004. Approves the National Pharmaceutical Assistance Policy. **Official Gazette of the Federative Republic of Brazil**, Executive Branch, Brasília, DF, 20 May. 2004. Section 1, p.52.

BRAZIL. Ministry of Health. **System for detecting psychoactive substance abuse and dependence: referral, brief intervention, social reintegration and follow-up, effects of psychoactive substances on the body.** 3. ed. Brasília, DF, 2006.

BRAZIL. Ordinance no. 344, of 12 May 1998. Approves the Technical Regulation on substances and medicines subject to special control. **Official Gazette of the Federative Republic of Brazil**, Executive Branch, Brasília, DF, 31 Dec. 1998.

Section 1, p.29.

BRAZIL. Resolution - National Health Council no. 466, of 12 December 2012. Approves regulatory standards for research involving human beings. **Diário Oficial [da] União**, Brasília, DF, 13 Jun. 2013d. Section 1, p. 59.

BRAZIL. Resolution - RE no. 1170, of 19 April 2006. List 1 - Form of Administration. Determines the publication of the guide for tests of relative bioavailability/bioquivalence of medicines. **Official Gazette of the Federative Republic of Brazil**, Executive Branch, Brasília, DF, 22 Apr. 2013c. Section 1, p. 101.

BRAZIL. Resolution - RE no. 1170, of 19 April 2006. List 2 - Analyses for Establishing Relative Bioavailability/Bioequivalence. Determines the publication of the guide for tests of relative bioavailability/bioequivalence of medicines. **Official Gazette of the Federative Republic of Brazil**, Executive Branch, Brasília, DF, 03 Aug. 2015. Section 1, p. 101.

BRAZIL. **Anxiety-related disorders**. 2008. Available at: http://www.datasus.gov.br/cid10/V2008/cid10.htm. Accessed on: 11 Sep. 2015.

CAMPIGOTTO, K. L. F. et al. Detection of the risk of interactions between antidepressants and associated drugs prescribed to adult patients. **Revista Psiquiatria Clínica**, v. 35, n. 1, p. 1-5, 2008.

CARVALHO, L. F.; DIMENSTEIN, M. The health care model and the use of anxiolytics among women. **Estudos de Psicologia**, v. 9, n. 1, p. 121-129, 2004.

CASTRO, G. L. G. et al. Use of benzodiazepines as self-medication: consequences of abusive use, dependence, pharmacovigilance and pharmacoepidemiology. **Revista Interdisciplinar**, v. 6, n. 1, p. 112-123, 2013.

CAVEDAL, L. E. **Quantification of clonazepam in human plasma by high-performance liquid chromatography coupled to mass spectrometer in a bioequivalence study**. 2014. 138 f. Dissertation (Master's in Medical Sciences) - State University of Campinas, Campinas, 2014.

CHAUHAN, B. L. et al. Comparative bioavailability study of clonazepam after oral administration of two tablet formulations. **Journal of the association of Physicians of India**, v. 48, n. 10, p. 985-987, 2000.

CHÈZE, M.; VILLAIN, M.; PÉPIN, G. Determination of bromazepam, clonazepam and metabolites after a single intake in urine and hair by LC-MS/MS. Application to forensic cases of drug facilitated crimes. **Forensic Sciense International**, v. 145, n. 2, p. 123-130, 2004.

COGHI, P. F.; COGHI, M. F. Stress and anxiety: are they eating you up? In: ISMA CONGRESS

ON STRESS, 14, 2013, Porto Alegre. **Proceedings...** Porto Alegre: ISMA, 2013. p. 1-13.

COSTA, E. M.; RABELO, A. R. M.; DE LIMA, J. G. Evaluation of the pharmacist's role in health promotion and disease prevention actions in primary care. **Revista de Ciências Farmacêuticas Básica e Aplicada**, v. 35, n. 1, p. 8188, 2014.

CREPALDI, L. B. **Analysis of medical records with an emphasis on diseases and their respective pharmacological treatments at the psychosocial care centre in a city in southern Santa Catarina - Criciúma.** 2013. 49f. Course Conclusion Work (Bachelor's Degree in Pharmacy) - Universidade do Extremo Sul Catarinense, Criciúma, 2013.

CRUZ, A. V. et al. Chronic use of diazepam in elderly people treated in the public health system in Tatuí-SP. **Revista de Ciências Farmacêuticas Básica e Aplicada**, v. 27, n. 3, p. 259-267, 2006.

DIÉYE, A. M. et al. Benzodiazepines prescription in Dakar: a study about prescribing habits and knowledge in general practitioners, neurologists and psychiatrists.
Fundamental & Clinical Pharmacology, v. 20, n. 3, p. 235-238, 2006.

DO AMARAL, B. D. A.; MACHADO, K. L. **Benzodiazepines: chronic use and dependence in Londrina - PR.** 2012. 31f. Course Conclusion Paper (Specialisation in Pharmacology) - Centro Universitário Filadélfia, Paraná, 2012.

FILHO, P. C. P. T. et al. Use of benzodiazepines by the elderly in a family health strategy: implications for nursing. **Escola de Enfermagem Anna Nery**, v. 15, n. 3, p. 581-586, 2011.

FIRMINO, K. F. et al. Use of benzodiazepines in the municipal health service of Coronel Fabriciano, Minas Gerais. **Ciência & Saúde Coletiva**, v. 17, n. 1, p. 157166, 2012.

FONSECA, A. L. **Interações medicamentosas.** 4. ed. São Paulo: EPUB, 2008.

FORMAN, S. A. et al. Principles of pharmacology of the central nervous system. p. 146 - 165. In: GOLAN, D. E. et al. (org). **Principles of pharmacology: the basis**

physiopathological pharmacotherapy. 3. ed. Rio de Janeiro: Guanabara Koogan, 2014.

GALLEGUILLOS, T. U. et al. Trends in the use of benzodiazepines in a sample of primary care consultants. **Revista Médica de Chile**, v. 131, n. 5, p. 535540, 2003.

GAVIN, R. S. **Depression, stress and anxiety: a focus on the mental health of workers - SP.** 2013. 109 f. Dissertation (Master of Science) - University of São Paulo, Ribeirão Preto, 2013.

GIL, A. C. **Como elaborar projetos de pesquisa**. 6. ed. São Paulo: Atlas, 2011.

GRAEFF, F. G. Anxiety, panic and the hypothalamic-pituitary-adrenal axis. **Revista Brasileira de Psiquiatria**, v. 29, supl.1, p. 53-56, 2007.

GREENBLATT, D. J. et al. Clonazepam pharmacokinetics: comparison of subcutaneous microsphere injection with multiple-dose oral administration. **Journal of Clinical Pharmacology**, v. 25, n. 11, p. 1288-1293, 2005.

HELOANI, J. R.; CAPITÂO, C. G. Mental health and work psychology. **São Paulo em Perspectiva**, v. 17, n. 2, p. 102-108, 2003.

HETEM, L. A. B.; GRAEFF, F. G. **Transtornos** de **ansiedade**. 2. ed. Rio de Janeiro: Atheneu, 2012.

HOCHMAN, B. et al. Research designs. **Acta Cirúrgica Brasileira**, v. 20, n. 2, p. 2-9, 2005.

HUF, G.; LOPES, C. S.; ROZENFELD, S. The prolonged use of benzodiazepines in women at a community centre for the elderly. **Caderno de Saúde Pública**. v. 16, n. 2, p. 351-362, 2000.

KOROLKOVAS, A.; BURCKHALTER, J. H. **Pharmaceutical Chemistry**. 5. ed. Rio de Janeiro: Guanabara Koogan, 2013.

LENZI, L.; GARCIA, C. G.; PONTAROLO, R. The pharmacist in SUS primary care. **Visão Acadêmica**, v. 12, n. 2, p. 55-64, 2011.

LOYOLA, A. I.; UCHOA, E.; LIMA, C. M. F Population-based epidemiological study on medication use among the elderly in the Metropolitan Region of Belo Horizonte, Minas Gerais, Brazil. **Caderno Saúde Pública**, v. 22, n.12, p. 26572667, 2006.

MANGINI, Z. A. **Conditioning factors related to the chronic use of clonazepam in Brazil: a life story -** SC. 2013. 91 f. Dissertation (Master's in Collective Health) - Federal University of Santa Catarina, Florianópolis, 2013.

MARCONI, M. A.; LAKATOS, E. M **Fundamentos de Metodologia Científica**. 7. ed. São Paulo: Atlas, 2010.

MARGONATO, F. B. As atribuições do farmacêutico na política nacional de medicamentos. **Infarma - Ciências Farmacêuticas**, v. 18, n. 3, p. 28-31, 2006.

MELO, O. F. et al. Knowledge and Practices of Pharmacists in the Multiprofessional Residency in

Family Health, Sobral - CE. **Revista de Políticas Públicas - Sobral**, v. 8, n.2, p. 16-25, 2009.

MENDONÇA, R. T.; CARVALHO, A. C. D. The consumption of benzodiazepines by elderly women. **Revista Eletrônica de Saúde Mental, Álcool e Drogas**, v. 1, n. 2, 2005.

MESTRINER, D. C. P. **O farmacêutico no serviço público de saúde: a experiência do Município de Ribeirão Preto** - SP. 2003. 124 f. Dissertation (Master's in Community Health) - University of São Paulo, Ribeirão Preto, 2003.

MIHIC, S. J.; HARRIS, R. A. Hypnotics and sedatives. p. 457- 479. In: BRUNTON, L. L.; CHABNER, B. A.; KNOLLMANN, B. C. (org). **The pharmacological bases of Goodman and Gilman's therapeutics**. 12. ed. Rio de Janeiro: Artmed, 2012.

MIYASAKA, L. S.; ATALLAH, A. N. Risk of drug clinical interactions: combination of antidepressants and other drugs. **Revista de Saúde Pública**, v. 37, n. 2, 2003.

MOTJABAI, R.; OLFSON, M. National trends in psychotropic medication polypharmacy in office-based psychiatry. **Archives of General Psychiatry**, v. 67, n. 1, p. 26-36, 2010.

MULULO, S. C. C. et al. Efficacy of cognitive and/or behavioural treatment for social anxiety disorder. **Revista de Psiquiatria do Rio Grande do Sul**, v. 31, n. 3, p. 177-186, 2009.

NOMURA, K. et al . Regular prescriptions for benzodiazepines: a cross-sectional study of outpatients at a university hospital. **Internal Medicine**, v. 45, n. 22, p. 12791283, 2006.

NORDON, D. G.; HUBNER, C. V. K. Prescription of benzodiazepines by general practitioners. **Diagnosis and treatment**, v. 14, n. 2, 2009.

NUNES, P. H. C. et al. Pharmaceutical intervention and prevention of adverse events. **Revista Brasileira de Ciências Farmacêuticas**, v. 44, n. 4, p. 691-699, 2008.

OLIVEIRA, A. B. et al. Obstacles to pharmaceutical care in Brazil. **Revista Brasileira de Ciências Farmacêuticas**, v. 41, n. 4, p. 409-413, 2005.

OLIVEIRA, L. C. F.; ASSIS, M. M. A.; BARBONI, A. R. Assistência farmacêutica no Sistema Único de Saúde: da política nacional de medicamentos à atenção básica à saúde. **Ciência & Saúde Coletiva**, v. 15, supl.3, p. 3561-3567, 2010.

ORLANDI, P.; NOTO, A. R. Misuse of benzodiazepines: a study with key informants in the municipality of São Paulo. **Revista Latino-Americana de Enfermagem**, v. 13, n. 13, p. 896-902, 2005.

RANG, H.P. et al. **Rang and Dale: Pharmacology**. 7. ed. Rio de Janeiro: Elsevier, 2011.

REIS, A. L. A. et al. **Pharmaceutical assistance for municipal managers**. Rio de Janeiro: PAHO/WHO, 2003.

REMINGTON, J.P. **A ciência e a prática da farmácia**. 20. ed. Rio de Janeiro: Guanabara Koogan, 2012.

SALLES, L. F.; SILVA, M. J. P. The identification of anxiety through iris analysis: a possibility. **Revista Gaúcha de Enfermagem**, v. 33, n. 1, p. 26-31, 2012.

SANTOS, H. C. et al. Possible drug interactions with psychotropic drugs found in patients from the East Zone of São Paulo. **Revista de Ciências Farmacêuticas Básica e Aplicada**, v. 30, n. 3, p. 285-289, 2009.

SEVERINO, A. J. **Metodologia do Trabalho Científico**. 23. ed. São Paulo: Cortez, 2007.

SILVA, P. **Farmacologia**. 8. ed. Rio de Janeiro: Guanabara Koogan, 2010.

SILVA, R. O.; BATISTA, M. L.; ASSIS, T. S. Analysis of the profile of benzodiazepine use in users of a university hospital in Paraíba. **Revista Brasileira de Farmácia**, v. 94, n. 1, p. 59-65, 2013.

DA SILVA, R. S. **Pharmaceutical care for the indiscriminate use of benzodiazepines - Rio de Janeiro**. 2012. 52f. Course Conclusion Paper (Bachelor's Degree in Pharmacy) - Centro Universitário Estadual da Zona Oeste, Rio de Janeiro, 2012.

SONG, D.; ZHANG, S.; KOHLHOF, K. Quantitative determination of clonazepam in plasma by gas chromatography-negative ion chemical ionisation mass spectrometry. **Journal of Chromatography**, v. 686, n. 2, p. 199-204, 1996.

SOUZA, L. E. P. F. Public health or collective health? **Espaço para a Saúde magazine**, v. 15, n. 4, p.07-21, 2014.

TREVOR, A. J.; WAY, W. L. Sedative - hypnotic drugs. p. 309 - 322. In: KATZUNG, B. G. (org). **Basic and clinical pharmacology**. 10. ed. Porto Alegre: AMGH, 2010.

TURATTI, M. E.; MARINI, D. C. Study of drug interactions in a psychiatric clinic in Mogi Guaçu. **FOCO: Caderno de Estudos e Pesquisas**, v. 5, n. 7, p. 11-30, 2014.

VIEIRA, F. S. Pharmaceutical assistance in the public health system in Brazil. **Revista**

Panamericana de Salud Pública, v. 27, n. 2, p. 149-156, 2010.

PREFEITURA DE SOBRAL
SECRETARIA DA SAÚDE
COMISSÃO CIENTÍFICA

PARECER PROTOCOLO Nº 0152/2015

Declaramos ter ciência dos objetivos e metodologia do projeto de TCC do Curso de Farmácia das Faculdades INTA intitulado: PERFIL DE USUÁRIOS DO MEDICAMENTO CLONAZEPAM DE UMA FARMÁCIA DA ESTRATÉGIA SAÚDE DA FAMÍLIA, desenvolvido por Crisliane Gomes de Amorim, sob orientação do Prof. Esp. Denilson Gomes Silva e co-orientaçao do prof. Dr. Cícero Igor Simões Moura Silva.

Na condição de instituição co-participante do projeto supracitado, concordamos em autorizar a realização da coleta de informações juntos às pessoas maiores de 18 anos que fazem uso regular de clonazepam, atendidas no Centro de Saúde da Família Maria Eglantine Ponte Guimarães, **desde que a abordagem seja realizada primeiramente por profissionais que indicarao aqueles que concordarem em participar do estudo e autorizarem acesso aos documentos solicitados.** Após esta etapa, será agendado os melhores dias e horários para realizaçao da coleta dos dados.

Ressaltamos que esta autorização NÃO desobriga os pesquisadores de solicitar anuência junto aos participantes, devendo estes serem convidados a participar mediante assinatura do Termo de Consentimento Livre e Esclarecido. Esta prerrogativa se baseia nas determinações éticas propostas na Resolução 466/2012 do Conselho Nacional de Saúde – CNS/MS, as quais, enquanto instituição co-participante, nos comprometemos a cumprir.

Esta autorização está condicionada à aprovação prévia da pesquisa supracitada por um Comitê de Ética em Pesquisa. O descumprimento desse condicionamento assegura-nos o direito de retirar esta anuência a qualquer momento da pesquisa.

Lembramos ainda que é de responsabilidade da pesquisadora encaminhar a esta Comissão Científica cópia da pesquisa no prazo máximo de 30 dias após sua conclusão.

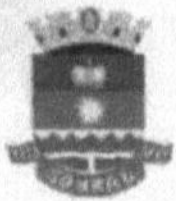

PREFEITURA DE SOBRAL
SECRETARIA DA SAÚDE
COMISSÃO CIENTÍFICA

Sobral, 13 de Janeiro de 2016

Profa. Dra. Maristela Inês Osawa Vasconcelos
Coordenadora da Comissão Científica

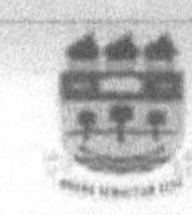 UNIVERSIDADE ESTADUAL
VALE DO ACARAÚ - UVA 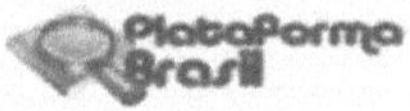

PARECER CONSUBSTANCIADO DO CEP

DADOS DA EMENDA

Título da Pesquisa: PERFIL DE USUÁRIOS DO MEDICAMENTO CLONAZEPAM DE UMA FARMÁCIA DA ESTRATÉGIA SAÚDE DA FAMÍLIA

Pesquisador: Denilson Gomes Silva

Área Temática:

Versão: 2

CAAE: 54222416.8.0000.5053

Instituição Proponente: INSTITUTO SUPERIOR DE TEOLOGIA APLICADA - INTA

Patrocinador Principal: Financiamento Próprio

DADOS DO PARECER

Número do Parecer: 1.579.536

Apresentação do Projeto:

O projeto faz parte do requisito parcial ao Curso de Bacharelado em Farmácia à Faculdade INTA - Instituto Superior de Teologia Aplicada, e consiste em analisar o Perfil de usuários do medicamento clonazepam de uma farmácia da Estratégia Saúde da Família. Trata-se de uma pesquisa de campo, descritiva, e também documental, exploratória, transversal e com uma abordagem predominantemente quantitativa.

Objetivo da Pesquisa:

Objetivo Primário:

Descrever o perfil de usuários do medicamento clonazepam de uma farmácia da Estratégia Saúde da Família.

Objetivo Secundário:

Identificar os usuários do clonazepam quanto ao sexo e idade; Buscar os tipos de associações com clonazepam nas prescrições ;Registrar o tempo de utilização do clonazepam pelos usuários; Analisar a origem das prescrições quanto à especialidade médica.

Endereço: Av Comandante Maurocélio Rocha Ponte, 150
Bairro: Derby   CEP: 62.041-040
UF: CE   Município: SOBRAL
Telefone: (88)3677-4255   Fax: (88)3677-4242   E-mail: uva_comitedeetica@hotmail.com

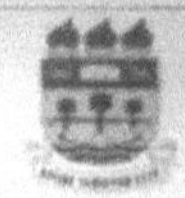

UNIVERSIDADE ESTADUAL
VALE DO ACARAÚ - UVA

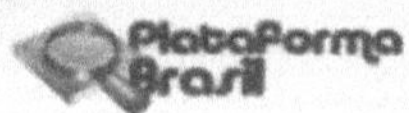

Avaliação dos Riscos e Benefícios:

Riscos informados:

Riscos mínimos e, para minimizar estes riscos, utilizará o manejo apenas de informações adquiridas por intermédio de um questionário com perguntas em que os participantes ficarão à vontade para responder, visando o sigilo e proteção dos mesmos. E, em seguida, o acesso das suas respectivas prescrições na farmácia do Centro de Saúde da Família.

Benefícios informados:

Os benefícios da pesquisa serão de identificar o número de usuário que utilizam o medicamento clonazepam cadastrados no local de estudo, auxiliar na adesão terapêutica e conduzir os usuários do sistema a progredir com o tratamento, por meio de acompanhamentos realizados pelo Farmacêutico e pela equipe multiprofissional.

Comentários e Considerações sobre a Pesquisa:

Pesquisa relevante para a área da Saúde Coletiva.

Considerações sobre os Termos de apresentação obrigatória:

Os termos encontram-se adequados.

Recomendações:

O projeto precisa ajustar o cronograma, visto que consta envio dos documentos ao CEP em março de 2016 e início da coleta dos dados em junho de 2016, porém só foi enviado ao CEP em maio de 2016, portanto a data de início da coleta dos dados precisa ser postergada.

Conclusões ou Pendências e Lista de Inadequações:

Ajustar cronograma.

Considerações Finais a critério do CEP:

O Colegiado do CEP/UVA, após apresentaçao e discussao do parecer pelo relator, acatou a relatoria que classifica como aprovado o protocolo de pesquisa. O(a) pesquisador(a) deverá atentar para as recomendaçoes listadas neste parecer.

Este parecer foi elaborado baseado nos documentos abaixo relacionados:

Tipo Documento	Arquivo	Postagem	Autor	Situação
Informações	PB_INFORMAÇÕES_BÁSICAS_710246	03/05/2016		Aceito

Endereço: Av Comandante Maurocélio Rocha Ponte, 150
Bairro: Derby   CEP: 62.041-040
UF: CE   Município: SOBRAL
Telefone: (88)3677-4255   Fax: (88)3677-4242   E-mail: uva_comitedeetica@hotmail.com

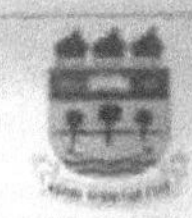 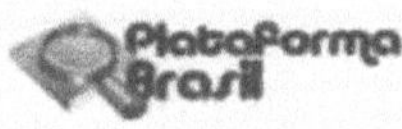

UNIVERSIDADE ESTADUAL
VALE DO ACARAÚ - UVA

Básicas do Projeto	E1.pdf	12:51:21		Aceito
Projeto Detalhado / Brochura Investigador	TCC_II_2016.pdf	13/03/2016 10:23:35	Denilson Gomes Silva	Aceito
TCLE / Termos de Assentimento / Justificativa de Ausência	APENDICE_B_TCLE_TCC.pdf	13/03/2016 10:18:55	Denilson Gomes Silva	Aceito
Outros	carta_de_anuencia.pdf	12/03/2016 00:13:31	Denilson Gomes Silva	Aceito
Orçamento	Orcamento_TCC.pdf	12/03/2016 00:06:12	Denilson Gomes Silva	Aceito
Cronograma	Cronograma_TCC.pdf	12/03/2016 00:03:42	Denilson Gomes Silva	Aceito
Folha de Rosto	Folha_de_rosto.pdf	11/03/2016 07:43:05	Denilson Gomes Silva	Aceito

Situação do Parecer:
Aprovado

Necessita Apreciação da CONEP:
Não

SOBRAL, 07 de Junho de 2016

Assinado por:
CIBELLY ALINY SIQUEIRA LIMA FREITAS
(Coordenador)

Endereço: Av Comandante Maurocélio Rocha Ponte, 150
Bairro: Derby   CEP: 62.041-040
UF: CE   Município: SOBRAL
Telefone: (88)3677-4255   Fax: (88)3677-4242   E-mail: uva_comitedeetica@hotmail.com

Research title: Profile of clonazepam users in a basic pharmacy of the family health strategy in the city of Sobral - CE.

Researcher: Crisliane Gomes de Amorim Lima

Supervisor: Prof°. Denilson Gomes Silva

You are being invited as a volunteer to take part in the research **"Profile of Clonazepam Users in a Basic Pharmacy of the Family Health Strategy in the City of Sobral - CE",** under the responsibility of the researcher Crisliane Gomes de Amorim Lima and the supervision of Professor Denilson Gomes Silva. In this study we intend to describe the profile of these users.

The reason for studying this subject could provide more significant information on the importance of correct therapy, in order to minimise unpleasant indices.

This research will use a quantitative approach, involving the preparation of documentation for data collection. A questionnaire and the prescriptions of 50 users of the drug clonazepam will be used. The researcher will treat their identity with professional standards of confidentiality.

The information obtained will be confidential and at any time that the FHSC user prefers not to take part or stops taking part in the study, this attitude will be understood by the researcher.

The results of the research will be made available to you when it is finalised. Your name or any material indicating your participation will not be released without your permission.

You will be guaranteed clarification and answers to any questions. If you have any questions, please contact the researcher Crisliane Gomes de Amorim Lima at the Instituto Superior de Teologia Aplicada - INTA, or on (88) 92737752.

If your questions are not resolved by the researcher, or your rights are denied, please contact the Research Ethics Committee of the Vale do Acaraú State University, located at the Health Sciences Centre (CCS), Avenida Comandante Maurocélio Rocha Ponte, 150, Campus do Derby, Sobral-CE, e-mail: CEP@uvanet.br, telephone: (88)3677-4255.

INFORMED CONSENT FORM

I ____ certify that after having received all the explanations and being aware of my rights from my supervisor Crisliane Gomes de Amorim Lima, I fully agree to the research being carried out. I therefore authorise the research work described above to be carried out with my spontaneous collaboration.

Sobral, 2016.

____

Participant's signature

Crisliane Gomes de Amorim Lima

Guidance student

Researcher responsible

APPENDIX B - DATA COLLECTION QUESTIONNAIRE

Research Title: Profile of Clonazepam Users in a Basic Pharmacy in the City of São Paulo Family Health Strategy in the city of Sobral - CE.

Researcher: Crisliane Gomes de Amorim Lima

Supervisor: Prof°. Denilson Gomes Silva

01. IDENTIFICATION DATA:

a. Sex: Female ( ) Male ( )

b. Age: _________

02. INFORMATION ON THE USE AND PURCHASE OF THE MEDICINE:

a. How long have you been taking clonazepam? _________________________________

b. What is the diagnosis for using the drug clonazepam?

____

c. Where did you go for your first appointment?

( ) In the CSF

( ) At CAPS

( ) In a public hospital

( ) In a private hospital

03. INFORMATION ON THE FIRST PRESCRIPTION:

a. Drug concentration ____

b. Posology___________________________

c. Are there any associated medication(s)? Which ones? _____________________________

d. Medical speciality _______________________________

e. The medicine is classified as: ( ) Reference; ( ) Generic; ( ) Similar.

42

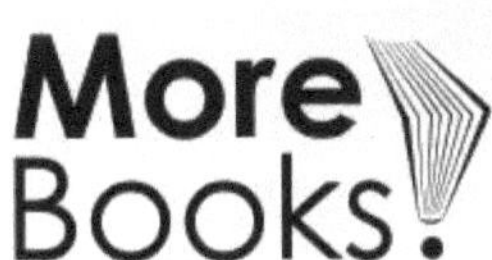

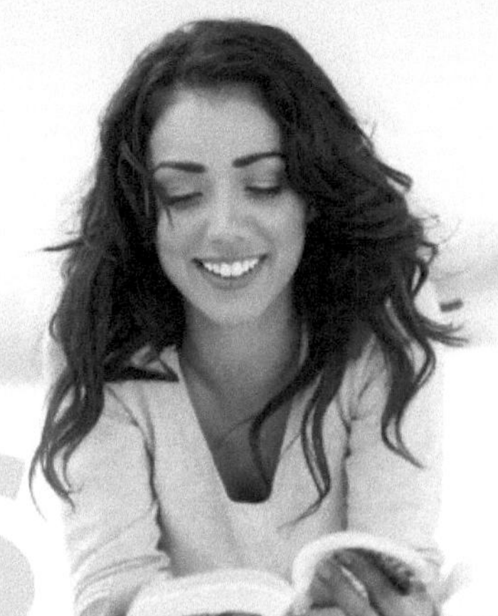

yes
I want morebooks!

Buy your books fast and straightforward online - at one of world's fastest growing online book stores! Environmentally sound due to Print-on-Demand technologies.

Buy your books online at
www.morebooks.shop

Kaufen Sie Ihre Bücher schnell und unkompliziert online – auf einer der am schnellsten wachsenden Buchhandelsplattformen weltweit! Dank Print-On-Demand umwelt- und ressourcenschonend produzi ert.

Bücher schneller online kaufen
www.morebooks.shop

info@omniscriptum.com
www.omniscriptum.com

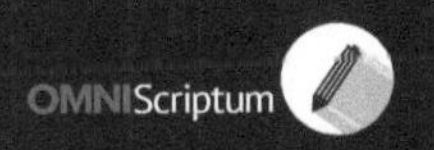

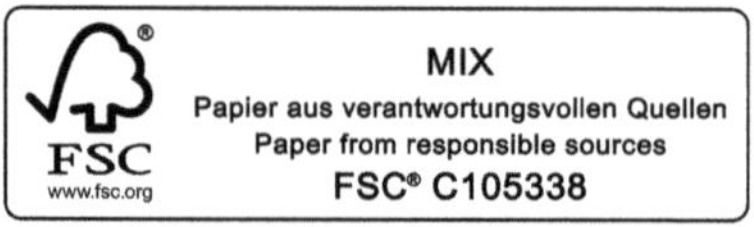

Printed by Books on Demand GmbH, Norderstedt / Germany